ESSENTIAL OILS

FOR WEIGHT LOSS

If You Are Not Using These Essential Oils You Are
Missing Out On Weight Loss Success

SOPHIE HART

Bonus: Download my Free E-book

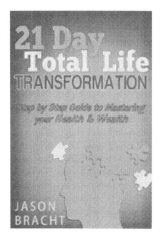

I have written an E-Book that I believe will help anyone who wants to make a lasting change in their life. The title is 21 Day Total Life Transformation. All you have to do is go to JasonBracht.com enter your email address and I will deliver it directly to your inbox.

This resource will help you get the most out of life – I lay out step by step techniques that can help dig you out of any rut.

To get instant access to these incredible tools and resources, click the link below:

Click here for the FREE 21 Day Total Life Transformation Book

ESSENTIAL OILS FOR WEIGHT LOSS

CONTENTS

INTRODUCTION

The term "essential oil" has been derived from the original word "quintessential oil." Now, here's a little history of the nomenclature:

In ancient times, it was thought that all matter is composed of four elements – water, earth, air and fire. Quintessence, or the fifth element, was regarded as the life force or the spirit at that time. It was considered as extremely important to remove this spirit from the plants. Therefore, specific processes were deployed to achieve this task. These included distillation and evaporation.

This also explains why the term 'spirit' is used for alcoholic beverages such as brandy, whiskey and eau de vie. In reality, this only meant 'the process of removal of the life force from the plant.'

Today, it is believed that essential oils do not hold any relevance to being spirits; they are physical in nature and are made up of complex mixtures of chemicals.

"The International Organization for Standardization (ISO) in their Vocabulary of Natural Materials (ISO/D1S9235.2) defines an essential oil as a product made by distillation with either water or steam or by mechanical processing of citrus rinds or by dry distillation of natural materials. Following the distillation, the essential oil is physically separated from the water phase."

It is extremely important for an essential oil to be separated by physical means only. The physical methods deployed in the process are distillation (these include steam, water and steam/water) or expression (also termed as cold pressing which is a feature unique to citrus peel oils). Maceration is another method deployed to create a few essential oils. This process involves maceration of the plant material in warm water with an aim of releasing the enzyme-bound essential oil. Examples of some of the essential oils produced through maceration are wintergreen, garlic, onion, bitter almond, etc.

Seems a little complex, correct?

Well, let me try and simplify this a bit. In simpler terms, essential oils are defined as liquids that are usually distilled from the leaves, stem, roots, bark, flowers or other parts of a plant. And here is a myth buster: essential oils do not have an oily feel! Surprised? Aren't you? Most essential oils are clear, however, some may be yellow or amber in color.

The true essence of the plants that are used in the process of extracting an essential oil is present in the oil that is extracted. These oils are really concentrated and just a little quantity will generally do the trick.

Is there a difference between essential oils and fixed oils?

Absolutely, unlike the fixed oils such as the olive oil, the essential oils are extremely volatile. They evaporate if left open.

Did you know that essential oils have been used since time immemorial to heal people? They provide the body with definite physical and mental benefits.

And now, here is another interesting fact:

Essential oils are used today to do much more work than just healing your body and mind. They can help you lose weight!

Yes, that's correct. Essential oils can aid in weight loss.

I know what you are thinking - Essential oils - weight loss? Where is the connection? How is this possible?

Let me now explain the science behind this:

Just imagine yourself walking past a coffee shop and experiencing the aroma of those freshly baked choco-chip muffins. You love the aroma, don't you? And now, your brain guides you to indulge yourself. You just want to eat those, correct? And you are not even sure of how they will taste - yet, the aroma works its magic!

Now, here is another question - Has it ever happened that you smelled some food and did not feel like consuming it? The smell of the food sent a message to your brain - hey, don't consume it! And the magic of aroma works yet again - you are not sure of the taste in this case as well, are you?

Now, a number of people associate hunger with blood sugar levels or 'a feeling of feeling full'. So, the thought process is - If you feel full, you are satiated! This is incorrect. The feeling of satisfaction or satiety is actually regulated by the satiety center in your hypothalamus (part of the brain). You stop consuming food because your satiety center sends a signal to you - hey, you are full now!

And can you influence this satiety center?

Absolutely! This can be influenced through your nose. The reason for this is that your nose is directly connected to your hypothalamus. Therefore, it can influence the satiety center in your hypothalamus. And that is the reason why certain aromas make you want more food and some make you repel food. Another important factor to be considered is that odor of things around you is sometimes intensified due to various other factors. And these factors then become important determinants in influencing your satiety center. The result? You either consume more food than you should be consuming or you begin to feel satiated without consuming food. Therefore, a direct connection between consumption of the amount of food and the odor around you is established.

You may want to test this by a simple activity. Walk past that chocolate doughnut counter and before you reach out to pick up your favorite doughnut, just take out your bottle of vanilla essential oil and smell it. This will almost instantaneously make you feel good and secure, thereby eliminating the need to consume that doughnut.

There are proven studies that indicate that smells such as basil, oregano and lemon can substantially diminish your appetite. In fact, inhaling these scents in each nostril for around six times can result in complete elimination of the desire to eat at that time. The flip side to this is that if you smell these scents only superficially, you may be tempted to eat more! Therefore, it is advisable to smell these scents as deeply as possible. It is also recommended that you change the scents that you smell frequently. This is because smelling a particular scent every day can lead to a feeling of deprivation which is the most common reason for failing to follow a particular diet.

What are the recommended scents?

Well, a number of individuals prefer sweet smelling scents such as green apple, chocolate or peppermint. These sweet smelling scents elevate the level of serotonin in your brain. Since serotonin is directly associated with cravings for sugar, you may see a marked reduction in your sugar consumption when you trigger this happy hormone via sweet smelling scents.

The book contains certain blend recipes that you can create at home. Carrier oils such as sweet almond, extra virgin coconut, walnut, grape seed, extra virgin olive oil etc. are used. In case you do not have the carrier oil that is suggested in the recipe, you may substitute with any other carrier oil of your choice. You must avoid certain oils such as walnut, coconut, almond etc. in case you suffer from nut allergies. Once again, substitution comes in handy here. Grape seed oil is the carrier oil of choice for all blends because it does not lead to any allergies.

ESSENTIAL OILS TO TRIM YOUR WAIST

Certain scents can actually trigger weight loss by directly influencing the capability of your body to burn fat. Some people notice a marked reduction in their waistline by consistent use of essential oil massage. Grapefruit, cypress and lemon oils are generally used for this purpose.

Now, before you start getting thoughts about an essential oil massage for ten days and a trimmed waistline.... Let me bring you back into the real world. While essential oils are great companions to your weight loss program, just essential oils are not enough! Your regular schedule of a healthy diet and appropriate exercise is extremely important in your weight loss journey.

ESSENTIAL OIL BLEND RECIPES FOR WEIGHT LOSS:

Blend recipe#1

A blend of Lavender, Basil, Grapefruit and Cypress with a carrier oil yields an ointment that is known to diminish or emulsify the fat present in the body. Sweet almond oil can serve as an excellent carrier oil. An aromatic bath or a full body massage is generally recommended.

Blend recipe#2

To prepare this blend, mix five drops each of lemon, grapefruit and cypress oils with 2ounces of sweet almond oil (which serves as the carrier oil). Blend everything together by pouring all these oils into a glass bottle and then rolling the bottle into your palms. (Ensure that the bottle is sealed at this time). You can begin by massaging this blend over your abdomen at least once in two days. Gradually, increase the frequency to once every day. Five times a week is the minimum recommended frequency.

This blend should not be exposed to sunlight since lemon and grapefruit may lead to photosensitivity. If you have accidently exposed this oil to sunlight, wait for around three hours before using it. Almost negligible allergic reactions have been observed with this oil. It is still recommended that you discontinue the use in case you notice any hives or rashes.

The recommended massaging technique is a circular oil massage. Massage your abdomen using outward strokes, starting from the belly button and using large circular strokes.

Blend recipe#3

This blend is made by mixing five drops each of fennel, juniper, cypress, rosemary and lemon essential oils with approximately one ounce of extra virgin coconut oil. Blend in a glass bottle and massage on your hips, thighs, belly and buttocks at least once every day. The technique used for massage is extremely important – outward large circular strokes!

Blend recipe#4

Seven drops of bergamot oil, twelve drops of fennel oil and five drops of patchouli oil are mixed with half an ounce of sunflower carrier oil. You can then blend the mixture thoroughly and use it to massage your abdomen several times in the day. Do not include the bergamot oil if you plan to be out in the sun right after the massage. This is because bergamot elevates the sensitivity of the skin towards the sun.

ESSENTIAL OILS FOR THAT NASTY FAT:

Lemon essential oil:

Lemon essential oil can definitely enable you to shed those pounds off your waist. The traditional uses of lemon include an elevated metabolism, improved circulation and an enhanced immune function. Lemon also curbs anxiety and helps in managing hypertension. The invigorating and warming aroma provides a great energy boost and demonstrates a proven antidepressant effect. It also promotes a general sense of wellbeing by bringing in more clarity and energy.

Lemon essential oil has been used since time immemorial to detoxify the body, boost metabolism, and stimulate secretions from pancreas, liver and stomach.

Consuming a drop of lemon essential oil mixed into a glassful of water is all it takes to achieve the perfect detoxification.

Around six to seven drops of lemon essential oil can be mixed with a tablespoon of extra virgin coconut oil. This can then be used to massage your abdomen, hips, thighs and buttocks. Massaging in outward, circular strokes will not only help you dissolve that nasty fat but also tighten your skin. Do not expose yourself to direct sunlight for at least twelve hours after the massage.

You may also use the lemon essential oil in the form of a capsule. You would only require a blank capsule (that can be easily sourced from your local chemist). Pour two drops of lemon essential oil and two drops of peppermint essential oil into the capsule. Next, add a few drops of extra virgin olive oil. Cover the capsule with its cap, shake well and consume with water – just the way you would consume any other oil. Isn't that the simplest way to lose weight?

Grapefruit essential oil:

Grapefruit, a proven diuretic possessing detoxifying properties, is refreshing and uplifting. It is an appetite suppressant that can diminish the number of fat cells. No wonder it is used in the treatment of cellulite!

A compound called citral is an important component of the grapefruit. Citral is known for its ability to curb appetite and stimulate metabolism. Research also proves that citral prevents the formation of new fat cells.

Want to control those cravings? Just inhale this oil to witness the magic. Cravings gone forever and all it takes is sixty seconds! Isn't that impressive?

Just add a drop of grapefruit essential oil to your bath to experience that ultimate relaxation and energy!

Mix five drops of grapefruit essential oil with a tablespoon of vegetable oil. Massage on the impacted areas. Regular use along with mild exercise and a healthy diet will ensure that you achieve the figure that you desire!

Pink grapefruit essential oil has a fruity aroma that can stimulate your senses and wake you up. Inhale this aroma frequently on the days when you are feeling low. Grapefruit essential oil inhaled at this time can help you reduce emotional eating.

Tired while working out? Just take out your grapefruit essential oil and inhale some. This will encourage you to get started once again. It does work on enhancing your motivation.

Mix five drops of grapefruit essential oil with three drops of basil essential oil and two drops of lemon essential oil. Massage your abdomen and hips with this blend in order to achieve that flawless complexion and figure.

Orange essential oil:

The orange essential oil is extracted from the peels of various kinds of oranges via the process of cold compression. Due to vast benefits that this oil brings, it is used in a number of products such as shampoos, soaps, body lotions and anti-aging solutions.

An excellent source of d-limonene, orange oil can support your body's natural cell repair process. It is excellent in clearing the toxins and helps in dissolving the fat located around the belly. The sweet aroma of this essential oil encourages relaxation and uplifts the mood.

You can mix around five drops of orange essential oil to a teaspoon of vegetable oil. Apply in firm, circular motion, using outward strokes over the abdomen.

You can also use this as a dietary supplement too! Never take any essential oil in its undiluted form. Always mix with a few drops of sweet almond oil, seal in a capsule and consume with water.

Fennel seed essential oil:

Fennel seed is often used as an alternative medicine remedy. The distinct flavor makes it useful for cooking purposes. It is an excellent source of magnesium, potassium, calcium and vitamins B and C. It is mainly used to heal gastrointestinal distress. The powerful antioxidant properties of fennel seeds help this essential oil to fight free radicals.

The fennel seed essential oil is extremely impactful when it comes to weight loss solutions. The positive impact may be attributed to its ability to facilitate the weight loss process as an appetite suppressant and a metabolic enhancer. The elevated metabolic output leads you to burn more energy and thus accelerates fat loss. Fennel also helps in breaking up the fat deposits present in the blood stream. These are used as energy. This in turn diminishes the cravings for foods.

Fennel also enhances the frequency of urination and diminishes water weight. This is especially useful in a scenario where a feeling of bloating is experienced due to retained water. The increased frequency of urination also leads to elimination of toxins from the body.

Massaging your body with fennel seed essential oil or consuming it in a capsule should definitely be a part of your weight loss strategy.

Some more essential oils:

Here are some more essential oils that must be a part of your weight loss kit:

- Rosemary
- Cedarwood
- Thyme
- Cumin
- Basil
- Fennel
- Geranium
- Lavender
- Oregano
- Patchouli
- Sage
- Spikenard
- Lime
- Juniper
- Cumin

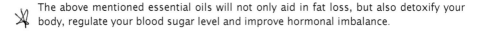 You can mix these with equal quantity of carrier oil (any good carrier oil such as any extra virgin oil) and massage it on to places that you term as 'problem areas' – could be places where that nasty fat accumulates (such as abdomen, hips, thighs, buttocks etc.). This should be done every day, at least two times in a day in case you want to witness visible results.

The above mentioned essential oils will not only aid in fat loss, but also detoxify your body, regulate your blood sugar level and improve hormonal imbalance.

ESSENTIAL OILS TO CURB THOSE CRAVINGS

Do you really want to lose weight? And you have made friends with essential oils that burn fat! WOW! However, did you know that in order to maintain your ideal weight, along with burning enough fat, it is extremely important to make alterations in your lifestyle that can enable you to control the calories that you consume? This means having a control over the portion size and managing your appetite.

Imagine you followed a grilling exercise schedule complemented by an essential oils massage every day for at least a month. Everybody is noticing your new look – your washboard abs and toned legs are grabbing eyeballs! Now, can you think of what would happen in case you started to eat whatever you wanted to (and this means quantity as well as quality)?

All the fat that you had previously burned would come back! Isn't that obvious? Yes, it is and it is equally scary! You don't want to be in that situation, correct? You really don't want to turn fat from fit – not again!

Okay, don't get so much bothered! We do have certain essential oils that can help you curb your appetite.

Lemon essential oil:

You learnt in the previous section about how lemon works on boosting your metabolism and burning fat. It has a profound detoxifying impact. It can also impact the area of your brain that guides you to eat more. You just have to smell the lemon essential oil to experience satiety and resist that urge to eat.

Peppermint essential oil:

This also helps in initiating a feeling of satiety. Just like the lemon essential oil, the peppermint essential oil impacts your hypothalamus and provides you a signal that you are already full. It is generally a good idea to inhale the aroma of peppermint essential oil just before meals. This ensures that you do not eat more than what you require and do feel satisfied with whatever you eat. You may even add two drops of peppermint essential oil into your evening tea. Isn't that the time when you feel the need to snack most?

Peppermint essential oil is a rich source of magnesium, potassium, iron, vitamin-C and omega-3 fatty acids. Using this as a part of your weight loss plan ensures that you are adequately nourished as you work towards losing weight. It is a great digestive aid too.

Another common method to use peppermint essential oil is by adding two drops into water or tea and consuming it just before your meal. This will ensure that you are able to resist that temptation for another serving of dessert.

Adding this oil to your bath water can enable you to feel full and refreshed!

Grapefruit essential oil:

We have already spoken about the many benefits of the grapefruit essential oil in the previous section. This is such a powerful oil for weight loss that it deserves a mention once again.

The grapefruit essential oil can enable you to curb your appetite. The digestive and diuretic properties of this oil can help your body to relieve water retention and dissolve fat.

Smelling grapefruit essential oil can enable you to curb your appetite whereas massaging it over the fat prone areas can help in burning body fat.

Ocotea essential oil:

The ocotea essential oil possesses a light cinnamon like aroma and flavor. It boasts of cleansing and purifying properties. Research indicates that this essential oil can diminish your cravings for food, lower your cortisol levels and help you manage your blood glucose levels too! It can even elevate your metabolism and liver functions. It is generally mixed with other essential oils that help to mask its strong aroma and enhance the benefits.

Five drops of ocotea essential oil is mixed with five drops of lemon essential oil and a tablespoon of extra virgin coconut oil. This creates a powerful fat burning blend that can be massaged on the impacted areas.

Two drops of ocotea essential oil in a cup of water should be consumed at least four times in a day. This acts as a very impactful appetite suppressant.

Some more essential oils:

It is well known that inhaling a scent regularly can help in diminishing appetite. The desire to eat is curbed by inhaling the aroma of these essential oils at least three to six times into each nostril. The desire to eat can also get enhanced if these oils are not smelled deeply. It is therefore extremely important that if you do decide to smell these oils, you smell them deeply!

Here are a few more essential oils that can help in suppression of appetite:

- Ylang-Ylang
- Clary-sage
- Rosemary
- Tangerine
- Vetiver
- Orange
- Patchouli
- Marjoram
- Cinnamon
- Spearmint
- Thyme
- Clove
- Fennel
- Wintergreen
- Patchouli

You should choose at least three essential oils that can be used during the day. Always carry these oils with you and rotate the oils that you use every day. So, if you are using Ocotea, grapefruit and fennel today, you may choose to use lemon, peppermint and marjoram tomorrow.

Now, take at least three to six whiffs in each nostril before each meal or whenever you feel the desire to eat something.

Do remember to close the cap tightly so that you do not unconsciously continue to inhale the aroma as this may decrease your sensitivity to essential oils.

Complete elimination of eating should not be your goal, and therefore overdoing this is not a great idea. You must just practice inhalation of essential oils in a manner that helps you take control of what you eat and when you eat.

ESSENTIAL OIL BLEND RECIPES TO CURB YOUR APPETITE:

You can use these blends whenever a craving comes along. You may want to use these in your kitchen, dining area, desk, coffee shop – or just anywhere. Always carry your bottle with you. Here are some blend recipes that can be used in order to curb those cravings:

- Forty drops of grapefruit essential oil, five drops of lemon essential oil and two drops of ylang ylang essential oil can be blended together in a glass bottle containing very little coarse sea salt.

- Thirty drops of peppermint essential oil, fifteen drops of bergamot essential oil, six drops of spearmint essential oil and one drop of ylang ylang essential oil can be blended in a glass bottle containing some coarse sea salt.

- Twenty drops of marjoram essential oil, twenty drops of basil essential oil, five drops of oregano essential oil and two drops of thyme essential oil can be blended in a glass water containing some coarse sea salt.

ESSENTIAL OILS TO ENHANCE THE WORK OUT

You do understand the importance of exercise, don't you? And if you have not begun your exercise regime yet, it's not too late to start now! Certain essential oils can profoundly elevate your motivation levels. Simply smelling, consuming and massaging these oils on your body can produce substantial results.

A number of athletes use essential oils to warm up their muscles and diminish the accumulated lactic acid after a strenuous exercise.

The most commonly used essential oils for working out are lavender, rosemary, eucalyptus, juniper berry, lemongrass, peppermint and sweet marjoram. Each essential oil, though used for work out has its distinct properties.

As an example the rosemary essential oil warms up muscles, relieves pain and boosts the mind and body. The lavender essential oil boasts of anti-inflammatory properties that help in pain relief, elimination of muscle spasms and also promotes mental calmness. Juniper berry essential oil eliminates the lactic acid from the muscles and also aids in the process of detoxification. Sweet marjoram eases the cramps in overworked muscles. The eucalyptus essential oil is invigorating and enhances circulation.

Essential oil blends can be created depending on the purpose they need to serve. The amount of essential oil used in the blend decides on how much energizing it will be. The greater the usage of essential oil, the better the stimulation. Prepare your oils based on your specific needs. So, if a more relaxing essential oil blend is required, use a higher concentration of carrier oil and lower concentration of essential oil. A combination of stimulating and relaxing can work well for your pre and post workout requirements.

Essential oils that can be used prior to the workout:

Getting to work out every day seems to be really hard for me. But not anymore! I have always been a person glued in front of the computer screen till 4:00pm. It was an obsessive compulsive disorder, I think! There were only two things that mattered to me – my laptop and my iPhone. I would insert reminders in my phone to remind me to work out. And yet, skip it! I would keep putting it off. And there were days when I would just not be able to push myself for a work out!

Today, the situation is different for me – working out is a totally painless experience for me and I am super motivated to kick start my work out every single day. The transformation came only because I got introduced to the fascinating world of essential oils. They energize me for my work out and are now an essential part of my gym bag.

You could actually create a blend of essential oils before you begin to work out. It is recommended that you add your essential oil to any lotion or water. Never apply pure essential oil onto your skin just before work out. This is because essential oils used in this manner may cause allergic reactions. Use of an aromatherapy diffuser is recommended.

How about an essential oil spray that fills you up with energy? Just add a few drops of peppermint, rosemary and eucalyptus essential oils into approximately two ounces of water. Mix them well and fill in a spray bottle. Spray on the exposed areas of the body at least thirty minutes prior to exercise. You can exercise once your skin has soaked up this essential oil blend. You don't want to sweat all the beneficial essential oils, do you? It is therefore recommended to use this spray at least thirty minutes prior to exercise.

Another essential oil blend can be prepared by mixing around twelve drops of rosemary essential oil, seven drops of eucalyptus essential oil and five drops of lavender essential oil into half an ounce of sweet almond oil. Massage it onto your skin at least half an hour before work out. This will warm up your muscles, enhance circulation, open your airways and awaken your mind.

It is recommended that you use a blend comprising of thirty drops of eucalyptus oil and one ounce of extra virgin coconut oil if you are suffering from asthma. Mix well and store in a dark colored glass bottle. Use this to massage your temples, neck and throat.

A blend comprising of five drops each of black pepper, peppermint, orange, lavender, geranium and rosemary essential oils in one ounce of grape seed oil can be massaged to soothe sore muscles. Stretch your muscles after the massage.

Inhaling peppermint essential oil prior to the work out can get you the motivation that you need.

It is extremely important to keep yourself hydrated prior to a workout. Increase your water intake at least two hours prior to a work out. Around six drops of lemongrass essential oil can be added to the water in order to enhance energy levels and alertness. Two drops of lemon essential oil in a glassful of water will not only enhance the flavor, but also super hydrate you. The oil is hydrating in itself and the aroma enhances the flavor of water, wanting you to drink more.

A blend of lemon, ocotea, spearmint, tangerine and grapefruit essential oil can energize your body, soothe sore muscles and elevate mental alertness and activity. Want to increase the thermogenic activity in the body? Add lemongrass essential oil to the blend! A compound named 'citral' is present in lemongrass essential oil. This enhances the thermogenic activity of the body.

Essential oils that can be used during a workout:

Essential oils are extremely useful during a workout session. A homemade essential oil workout spray can enhance skin clarity and energize your body. Always store your blends in dark colored glass bottles.

A water spray mister is one of the best ways to enjoy the advantages of a workout blend. Since water and essential oils do not mix very well, shake the bottle vigorously prior to use.

Fifteen drops of bergamot essential oil, eight drops of sage essential oil and ten drops of cypress essential oil can be mixed together and poured into a spray bottle along with a cup of pure distilled water. Feel free to spray this over the exposed areas of your skin in order to prevent it from breakouts. Don't forget to do a patch test prior to first use of this blend. A patch test is done by spraying a little quantity over a small area of the skin. You should not use the blend in case you experience any allergies, hives, itchy feeling, redness etc.

Muscle soreness can be addressed by frequent application of the blend followed by stretching of muscles.

Another blend recipe could be prepared by mixing five drops each of lavender, lemon, petitgrain, eucalyptus and rosemary essential oil. Use this as a spray on your skin during your workout. Once again, a patch test is recommended prior to use. Don't forget to cover your eyes before spraying this on your body as the oil could be dangerous for the eyes.

Keeping yourself hydrated during a workout is equally important. Two drops of lemon essential oil in a glassful of water sipped during the water is not only nourishing, but also hydrating and soothing.

Essential oils that can be used post a workout:

You do sweat during a workout, don't you? Always shower right after the workout. This will enable you to get rid of the dirt, sweat and bacteria. It will also soothe your muscles and diminish any inflammation.

You can use a blend of lemongrass, grapefruit, tangerine and coriander to wash off the dirt and refresh yourself. Apply lemongrass essential oil on your sore muscles right after you shower. This will help you eliminate inflammation and prepare you for the workout for the next day. Post this, apply tea tree essential oil onto your feet. The tea tree essential oil guards against fungus and bacterial infections.

Getting that feeling of soreness in the entire body? No problem, just mix some Epsom salt and lavender essential oil to your bath water and soak yourself up in the luxury of your tub. Now, that's what we call heaven on earth! Lavender essential oil aids in soothing sore knees, shoulders, ankles and back.

Another essential oil called Helichrysum italicum is effective in improving circulation and hastening the healing process. It is often termed as the 'everlasting oil' due to its excellent ability to heal the body. This is precisely the reason why this is often used for bruises. Eighty percent of this oil can be diluted with twenty percent of sweet almond or jojoba oil.

Eucalyptus essential oil works as an impactful after shower oil. Just mix thirty drops of eucalyptus essential oil, twenty drops of thyme oil and twenty drops of clove oil with an ounce of grape seed oil to form a soothing massage blend. Use this post the shower. A slight tingling sensation post usage is absolutely acceptable. You can substitute grape seed oil with extra virgin coconut oil or sweet almond oil. Be careful about the usage of oil in case of nut allergies. The massage technique to be deployed is long strokes moving towards the heart.

Another massage oil blend that can be used involves mixing six drops of juniper berry essential oil, six drops of ginger essential oil and ten drops of sweet marjoram essential oil. Dilute this in half an ounce of extra virgin olive oil and treat yourself to that relaxing bliss!

Around fifteen drops of eucalyptus essential oil, ten drops of peppermint essential oil and five drops of lavender essential oil can be mixed with an ounce of sweet almond oil to create a blend that works wonders for sore muscles.

Here are a few more blend recipes that can help to heal sore muscles:

- Eight drops of juniper berry essential oil, ten drops of lavender essential oil and five drops of lemon essential oil diluted with half an ounce of sunflower oil.

- Twenty drops of rosemary essential oil, ten drops of peppermint essential oil and ten drops of sweet marjoram essential oil can be diluted in one ounce of extra virgin olive oil to create a soothing blend that works like magic on tired and aching muscles.

Another simple remedy to treat muscle soreness is to soak yourself up in a hot water tub that contains a few drops of lavender, lemon and eucalyptus oil. Just sit in the tub for fifteen minutes and notice how your muscles thank you for taking care of them!

ESSENTIAL OILS THAT CAN HELP CURB EMOTIONAL EATING

Did you know that your emotional state directly influences the way you eat? You normally end up consuming a lot more food than what is required in case you are anxious, depressed, tired, angry or stressed. This is because subconsciously you want to fill up a void in your life. The easiest way to do this is via food because food instantaneously makes you feel better about yourself.

The aroma of essential oils has a direct impact on your endocrine system which influences the way you feel about things. They help you view yourself in a positive light and therefore provide that much needed boost to your mental health. This automatically diminishes your stress levels and elevates your mood.

So, the next time you feel like filling that void in your life, just reach out for that bottle of essential oil in your cupboard and inhale, bathe, massage – just use it to make you feel better about yourself and life!

Tangerine, rose geranium and bergamot are the most common essential oils that are used for this purpose. Bergamot is the recommended one amongst these owing to its unique property to relieve anxiety, stress and tension. The calming impact of this oil provides the much needed hormonal support. Want to experience real calmness? Just combine this with some lavender oil and use it in your bath! Isn't it pure bliss?

Rose geranium is extremely impactful in lifting your mood, detoxifying your body and creating a hormonal balance.

Tangerine is not only impactful in diminishing anxiety, but also helps in regulating metabolism and eliminating cellulite.

Here is the complete list of essential oils that can be used to beat stress:

- Lavender essential oil: This one is known for its antidepressant, relaxing and anti-inflammatory properties. It can treat insomnia, high blood pressure, tension induced headaches, anxiety and tachycardia.

- Patchouli essential oil: This one is great for balancing emotions and treating anxiety and depression. Just add it to your bath water, use it for your massage or inhale it via diffusers to experience the magic. This oil acts as a stimulant and energizes you if used in small quantities. It acts as a sedative and calms your nervous system if used in large quantities.

- Valerian root essential oil: Valerian root essential oil can be mixed with patchouli, pine or lavender essential oil to provide relief from indigestion, insomnia, migraine and anxiety.

- Chamomile essential oil: The calming and sedative impact of this oil plays a significant role in managing anxiety and depression. Do not use this remedy in the first and second trimester of pregnancy.

- Clary sage essential oil: This helps in diminishing symptoms of depression and anxiety such as insomnia and restlessness. Inhaling the vapors of this oil for fourteen consecutive days can help in eliminating symptoms of depression and anxiety.

- Tangerine essential oil: This is most used when you want to regulate your sleep patterns. It is calming, relaxing and sedative.

- Lemon balm essential oil: The lemon balm essential oil finds use as a sedative, hypnotic and antidepressant. It helps in reducing high blood pressure, relieves insomnia, stress, tension and calms the mind. You may combine it with ylang-ylang, neroli, lavender, lemon, geranium or bergamot to create a few interesting blends.

- Neroli essential oil: The neroli essential oil can elevate your mood, provide relief from depression, improve blood circulation and provide relief from stress and tension.

- Bay laurel essential oil: This one keeps those feelings of anxiety and melancholy at bay and aids in creating a greater mental balance. It can boost your self-esteem and eliminate those feelings of nervousness.

- Magnolia essential oil: One of the most impactful essential oils for relieving anxiety and tension, the magnolia essential oil truly relaxes the mind.

- Vetiver essential oil: This is used to calm a hyperactive mind and harmonize emotions. It can enable you to recover from any shock or mental trauma and hence cope up with stress.

- Basil essential oil: Truly stimulating and refreshing, the basil essential oil eases off mental fatigue quickly. An impactful relaxing blend can be created by mixing ten drops of basil essential oil, ten drops of bergamot essential oil, two drops of eucalyptus essential oil, five drops of lavender essential oil and five drops of peppermint essential oil.

- Eucalyptus essential oil: The eucalyptus essential oil blends very well with grapefruit, ginger, cypress, chamomile, marjoram, lavender, juniper, rosemary, pine, peppermint and thyme essential oils. It enables you to combat extreme fatigue, stress, anxiety, depression and headaches.

- Coriander essential oil: This has a real uplifting impact and helps in diminishing all worries. It also fights anxiety, mental fatigue, depression and stress. It blends beautifully with cinnamon, grapefruit, ginger, neroli, lemon and bergamot essential oils.

- Geranium essential oil: A nervous tonic that helps in relieving depression, anxiety and stress, this one truly relaxes and reenergizes you.

- Bergamot essential oil: The bergamot essential oil reduces anxiety, fear, anger and stress. It not only diminishes your mental tensions, but works on eliminating your physical tensions too!

- Lemon essential oil: The lemon essential oil enables you to make swift decisions, helps in clarifying ideas and eliminates your worries. Use four drops in a diffuser or around fifteen drops in bath water as a quick fix to anxiety.

- Lime essential oil: The lime essential oil reenergizes the body and reduces depression, anxiety and exhaustion. You can create interesting blends by mixing a few drops of lime essential oil with equal quantities of lavender or clary sage essential oils.

- Spikenard essential oil: This is the essential oil of choice to promote a Zen state and establish inner peace and harmony. Massaging with this oil can enable you to treat insomnia, anxiety and headaches

- Jasmine essential oil: Jasmine essential oil is used in aromatherapy to relax the nerves, eliminate anxiety and fear, treat depression and restore energy. It blends extremely well with ylang-ylang, rose, neroli and lavender essential oils.

- Frankincense essential oil: It soothes the nervous system and diminishes fear and anxiety.

HOW TO USE ESSENTIAL OILS FOR WEIGHT LOSS?

Here are the different ways to use these essential oils in order to provide you with maximum health and healing:

Inhalations: Inhalations can be accomplished by using essential oils in diffusers, hot compresses or in hot water. The recommended dose is generally ten drops and this is the most preferred and impactful method to use these oils. To facilitate the process of steam inhalation, around seven drops of essential oil are added to two cups of boiling water. The steam is then inhaled via nose by placing the nose at around twelve inches from the bowl containing the water.

Diffusers: You may also use an oil burner. All you need to do is add around ten drops of oil to two tablespoons of warm water and light the candle after placing the mixture in the burner bowl. Within a few minutes, you would notice your room filling up with the aroma of these oils.

Bath: Some people prefer using these essential oils in their bath. If you are one of those, then you may use ten drops of your chosen essential oil with a tablespoon of milk to your bath water. The milk acts are a carrier and prevents your skin from burning.

Massage: An essential oil massage can do a ton of good to your mind and body. Once again, don't forget to use your carrier oil. The ideal proportion is five milliliters of carrier oil for three drops of essential oil. Sweet almond oil and grape seed oil are recommended for usage.

Cloth: You may inhale the pleasant aroma of essential oils via your pillow or handkerchief. Just place four drops of oil on your pillow before you prepare to sleep. The scent from this will help you sleep better. Likewise, inhalation via handkerchief can almost instantly uplift your mood.

IMPORTANT DO'S AND DON'TS FOR ESSENTIAL OILS:

Here are some Do's and Don'ts about essential oils:

Do's:

- Educate yourself: You must educate yourself about the various uses of essential oils. It is always a good idea to familiarize yourself with shopping guides about essential oils and also the safety instructions related to them.

- Shop wisely: You should always shop from trusted shops or brands. A number of times manufacturers claim that their essential oils are pure and undiluted. However, this may not be the case. You must research for the brand that provides highest quality essential oils as this may vary from one brand to another.

- Read all relevant information: This may include the methods of extraction, botanical name of the oil, the country of origin and even the method of farming. This way, it can be ascertained if the oil is organic or not.

- Store appropriately: Store your oils in dark colored glass bottles (cobalt blue or amber) and in a cool and a dark place.

- Safety comes first: Yes, read and pledge to follow all safety precautions before starting to use an oil.

- Enjoy yourself! If you have decided to embrace aromatherapy and essential oils for weight loss, make it a point to enjoy the experience. Pamper yourself to your favorite indulgences, complement these with a consistent exercise schedule and a balanced nutritious diet and you would notice that the oils begin to work their magic on you.

Don't's :

Don't confuse essential oils with perfume oils: These are two entirely different things. Perfume oils can never offer the same advantages as essential oils.

Don't compromise on the packaging: Be extremely careful about the manner in which your oils are packaged. Some manufacturers sell essential oils with rubber glass marker tubes. The concentration of the essential oils can convert these rubber tubes into gummy structures, spoiling the oil.

Don't ever compare apples to oranges: Some common plants used to create essential oils are Eucalyptus, Anise, Bay and Cedarwood. However, a number of essential oils can be obtained from the various varieties available for each of these plants. And all these may be priced differently. It would be a good idea to look at the botanical names for the plants used in the extraction of these essential oils. An example here could be the 'Bay essential oil'. The essential oil from Pimenta racemosa is used to prepare this oil. Similarly, this oil is also prepares from the plant, Laurus nobilis.

Do not purchase your oils from craft shows or street fair: Yes, never do it! These may be low on quality and you may never be able to find the same seller again! Most reputed manufacturers do not sell their oils in one-time events or shows.

SAFETY WITH ESSENTIAL OILS

This is an extremely important topic. It must be understood that essential oils are extremely harmful if they are not used with caution. Here are the recommended safety guidelines:

- Always use essential oils in their diluted form. The undiluted ones may sometimes cause serious allergies or reactions.

- Always check the sensitization reaction of the essential oil via skin patch tests. Just place two drops of diluted essential oil on the inside of your elbow and cover it with a bandage. This area must not get wet for the next twenty four hours. Essential oils are safe for use in a scenario where you do not experience any irritation. However, if you do experience any irritation, you should consider removing the bandage and washing the area with soap and water. Do not use this essential oil now because your patch test has proved that you are sensitive to this oil.

- Each essential oil has a definite set of safety precautions associated with it. Do make an effort to familiarize yourself with the safety precautions of the oil that you are using, especially if you suffer from some specific health conditions such as asthma, allergy or even pregnancy.

- Essential oils are extremely powerful. Always use the recommended smallest possible amount. If the recommended dosage is two drops, do not go overboard and use three.

- Essential oils should almost never be consumed internally (the only exception to this rule is a recommendation from your aroma therapist detailing the steps to use the oil).

- Essential oils should not be used by children, except under adult supervision. The fragrant smell of essential oils may attract kids towards them. However, it should be noted that these oils are miraculous when used with caution and can serve as fatal when used without proper knowledge.

- Some essential oils are phototoxic and should not be applied to skin that will be directly exposed to sunlight in the next twenty four to thirty six hours. These include Petitgrain, Bergamot and Citrus oils.

- Essential oils can sometimes react with toxins that have accumulated in the body as a result of chemicals in water, food or general environment. It is recommended to stop the usage of these oils in case you experience a reaction due to a build-up of toxins. Also increase your water intake when you start with essential oil therapy.

- Sustained exposure to essential oils during massage sessions can lead to feelings of headaches, vomiting's, nausea and general uneasiness. Therapists should therefore ensure proper ventilation, frequent breaks and adequate amount of water. Operating any kind of motorized equipment should be avoided post usage of certain essential oils. Examples of these are clary or sage. A week's rest is generally advised post two weeks of essential oil usage.

DILUTING YOUR ESSENTIAL OILS

A number of people claim that it is safe to use Lavender oil and Tea tree oil in skin without dilution. In fact, they insist that some essential oils are extremely beneficial when applied 'neat'.

Applying neat implies applying an essential oil without any dilution. Now, this can be extremely dangerous. In fact, the oils that you think can be applied neat (Lavender oil and Tea tree oil) also should not be used directly on the skin. This is because undiluted oils may lead to a permanent sensitization reaction on your skin. You definitely don't want these, correct?

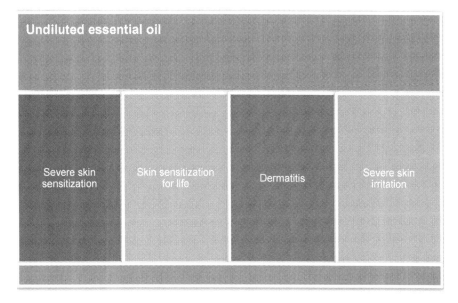

Diluting essential oils enables you to save some money along with ensuring your well-being.

A two percent solution of an essential oil is considered safe in case you want to utilize it for adult topical application. Elderly and children can do with one percent solution.

The market is flooded with highly fragrant and scented synthetic products such as shampoos, oils, perfumes, deodorants, toners, face washes, body lotions etc. A two percent dilution therefore may seem to be really weak in the beginning. However, over time, you will accustom yourself to the new natural science of scent and start savoring the shades of your diluted oils.

An easiest method used for creating your two percent dilution is to use twelve drops of essential oil and thirty ml. of any cold pressed carrier oil such as sweet almond oil, pomegranate seed oil, peanut oil, jojoba oil and hazelnut oil.

The dropper method is not the most accurate method, primarily because of the difference in the size of drops of various essential oils. This difference in size may result from the difference in the size of the dropper, the viscosity of the oil or the temperature of the oil. However, it is considered the most acceptable methods while working with small quantities of oil.

THE DILEMMA OF SUBSTITUTION

Well, quite often you may be faced with the dilemma of substitution. You may want to create an essential oil blend and just not have the exact recommendation available with you. In this scenario, you can carefully substitute the recommended oil with one of the essential oils that you already possess. You just have to clear about the purpose of substitution. So, if you do not possess an essential oil that can help you manage stress, you can substitute with any other oil that has somewhat similar properties. Be very careful to read the safety precautions first.

I hope that I have been able to empower you with enough information about essential oils and how you can specifically use them for weight loss. Now is the time to start applying all this information and making essential oils an important part of your weight loss journey. Consistent exercise, balanced and nutritious meals and optimum usage of essential oils can get you the dream body that you desire. Use this book as your companion or guide in order to enter the fascinating world of essential oils and experience ultimate weight loss and cellulite reduction! All the best!

Thank You

Before you go, I want to warmly say "thank you" from the bottom of my heart! I realize that there are many e-books on the market and you decided to purchase this one so I am forever grateful for that.

Thanks a million for reading this book all the way to very end!

If you enjoyed this book then I need your help!

Please take a moment to leave a review for this book after you turn the page.

This valuable feedback will allow me to write e-books that help you in your journey through life. And if you love it, please let me know.

40734150R00020

Made in the USA
Lexington, KY
16 April 2015